WAKE UP

Design YOUR Focus:

UNDERSTAND THE POWER YOU HAVE WITHIN TO
CONNECT YOUR LIFESTYLE WITH YOUR
EMOTIONS, HEALTH AND RELATIONSHIPS

DEANA PATTERSON, MBA, CMR, BCCL

WAKE UP Design YOUR Focus Book is available at special quantity discounts for bulk purchase for sales promotions, premiums, fund-raising, and educational needs. For details email www.deanapatterson@dsfit2run.com

To contact the author, visit
WEBSITE: www.thehealthandfitnessadvocate.com

ISBN- 13: 978-1542774819

ISBN- 10: 1542774810

Printed in the United States of America

DEDICATION

This book was inspired by my life experiences and struggles to improve my mind, body and soul for a complete Lifestyle balance.

My Health Coaching experience at the Institute for Integrative Nutrition (IIN), where I received my training in holistic wellness and health coaching.

IIN offers a truly comprehensive Health Coach Training Program that invites students to deeply explore the things that are most nourishing to them. From the physical aspects of nutrition and eating wholesome foods that work best for each individual, to the concept of Primary Food – the idea that everything in life, including our spirituality, career, relationships, and fitness contributes to our inner and outer health – IIN helped me reach optimal health and balance. This inner journey unleashed the passion that compels me to share what I've learned and inspire others.

Beyond personal health, IIN offers training in health coaching, as well as business and marketing. Students who choose to pursue this field professionally complete the program equipped with the communication skills and branding knowledge they need to create a fulfilling career encouraging and supporting others in reaching their own health goals.

From renowned wellness experts as Visiting Teachers to the convenience of their online learning platform, this school has changed my life, and I believe it will do the same for you. I invite you to learn more about the Institute for Integrative Nutrition and explore how the Health Coach Training Program can help you transform your life. Feel free to browse my website and contact me to hear more about my personal experience at

http://www.thehealthandfitnessadvocate.com or

http://geti.in/1JtssPh or call (844) 315-8546 to learn more.

This book is dedicated to the memory of my mom, Charlotte Victoria Simmons for my actual birth leading to our spiritual connection, the growth of knowledge, and consistent courage to birth my first book. I miss you everyday, but I talk to you daily with a smile on my face and happiness in my heart.

And to

My amazing Daughter Brittanie Danielle Russell for your Love and Support and always believing in your mother. I love your demeanor and positivity as you grow to understand the reasoning behind my discipline as a single parent and to maturing as my best friend.

I LOVE YOU!!!!!

CONTENTS

ACKNOWLEDMENTS

ACKNOWLEDGMENTS

To my daughter Brittanie, the gift from God that allows my love, joy and happiness to blossom everyday. You are such a treasure and a brightness to my heart. I am grateful for your love and support.

To Mr. Pugh, thank you for your continuous support, spiritual guidance and your fatherly advice.

To my DSFIT2RUN members, thank you for the continuous discussion on our weekend walks and discovering our healthy journey along the way.

To my Family, thank you for allowing me the time to dig deep internally and improve my actions by focusing on my inner spiritual growth.

To my dear friends Tashra, Angela and Angie, thank you for your continuous prayers, positive encouragement, and always allowing my return to the ultimate spiritual center after each conversation.

To my Sisters, we are blessed to have a second chance to create a loving sister bond that will last a lifetime!!! Love you Divas

To Dr. Abdul Sankari thank you for your friendship and encouragement with every visit as well as your clinical feedback providing a great balance.

To Dr. Joseph Stella, thank you for your consistent friendship and honest feedback with every visit. I appreciate your listening ear and positive attitude.

To Gloria my prayer warrior, thank you for your friendship and consistent support. This helps me stay focused with my Faith in God, which confirms my passion, dedication, and purpose to Wake UP and Design my Focus.

CHAPTER 1

INTRO - DO YOU LISTEN

IT IS OUR RESPONSIBILITY to be in love with ourselves to be the best expression of vitality, health, and well being that we can possibly be to honor ourselves. If we want to activate change, we cannot worry about what others think of us, but how we will be responsible for ourselves. We have to always be present and live in the now. Thereby, allowing you to choose to love yourself, trust the future and what's to come. We get upset when things do not go according to plan, but we have to realize that this is not our plan. Remember, when the plan goes another way, get excited because you should know you are a step away from a breakthrough or what I like to say is a huge transformation. I believe if you are willing to see it, believe it, dream it, speak it, and stay consistent with your faith, you can bring it into existence. Stop looking at things through the lens of a victim or the glass being half full because it will keep you in the victim's position. Your life will not always go as planned because if you expect it to be 100% predictable, you will end up in a vicious circle. Your experiences will stay within the same atmosphere keeping you in a negative outcome over and over.

DO YOU LISTEN

Let's be a student of life with maintaining Trust & Faith to gain knowledge from the past experiences allowing you to grow into your future and benefit from your past. You will then be able to answer the questions that are on your mind:

Why is this happening to me?

What did I do to deserve this problem?

Why?

Is this my lesson or a future problem for someone in my life?

Am I helping someone else get through?

Reflect on your answer:

_____

_____

_____

_____

_____

So, let's start focusing on what we want because sometimes it's a process of elimination before we really step into understanding our true internal self. When you discover your true inner self, it should connect you to a nutritional journey that should lead you to a healthy lifestyle.

The question becomes, at what age do you really know the true you? We go through life always questioning our actions to be our worst critic. I have only met a few people in my life that truly live for the moment with no cares or worries in the world. I honestly would always judge them because my perception was they have no sense of time (always late), and I always thought they didn't really care about others because it was always about them. They always wanted situations to go their way and never really took true ownership of faults, mistakes or life lessons.

Again, this is my opinion, but now that I am a little older and wiser, I can definitely see they were just living in the now and making sure that happiness was on the top of the list or, should I say, Self-love?

This brings me back to flying. Remember when you are on the plane, and they instruct you in an emergency to put your oxygen mask on first because you need to be in control to allow yourself to help others. Life has to be the same allowing you to focus on the best you to make sure that you can then assist others to be their best. The results will have a ripple effect allowing for success stories all over the world. Each one teaches one to make a better world allowing you to give back to help others that may be experiencing your past issues. You will be their lifesaver to help them transition into a better situation. You will learn to let go of some people in your lives on the way to discovering the real you. So the next time your expectations don't match your reality, instead of asking "Why?" because you may never really know the answer. Just ask yourself the following questions:

What is my lesson?

How can I not repeat this situation?

What will I need to do to grow from this situation?

Reflect on your answer:

_____

_____

_____

_____

_____

Trust me; you will feel fulfilled because this will allow you to start loving yourself or what I call self-motivation. You do this by focusing and visioning what you want to become, experience, and how you want to feel. You have that inner voice inside, some call it a spirit and others say God is talking to them. Whatever you believe, listen to it, as it will always lead you in the right direction.

The first step is to listen and be obedient to the guidance. Have the courage to listen to your inner self because I am just now really focusing and getting it as I write my 1st book. This journey is allowing me to dig deeper and realize my issues that need to be addressed. I now understand that I have to let go and be free in order to love myself and love my future experiences. I am starting to really take time alone and truly listen to my inner voice allowing me to be first. This is definitely taking time because I have always put everyone first and left me for last. I now understand my actions toward others and the reasons that I just don't want to tolerate the treatment from others.

The problem that I am discovering is that the treatment has been around for years and now I am designing my focus to have pure happiness in my life. Now, don't get me wrong, I have always purchased the items that I desired, gone on vacations and outings from time to time. I am talking about really getting to know the true self, getting away from the material lifestyle and finding out what's really bothering me.

I know that I can be my own worst critic and I struggle with forgiveness, but I now understand that if I wipe the slate clean, I allow room for my blessings. So now I ask myself, is it deeply rooted with my family disconnections or what's really holding me back? This book will allow doors to be opened, questions to be answered, and dreams to be fulfilled. You will be able to cancel negativity out of your life. You will be able to grant forgiveness, love for others, and self-love to design your new focus.

My friend Tashra believes that you cannot lose your peacefulness through others' madness. Learn to find happiness and joy every day. I believe that if you stay true to your inner self this will allow you to focus on a better you. I love the message from Joel Osteen as follows, "You need to expect unprecedented favor to unlock the promises over your life."

I am a certified Health coach, a pharmaceutical sales representative and owner of DSFIT2RUN, nonprofit organization. I have studied in the health field for many years, and it has increased my desire to help others cultivate a healthy journey with an understanding that this is a lifestyle. I received my Health Coach training from the Institute for Integrative Nutrition, where I studied a variety of dietary theories and practical lifestyle coaching methods. When you agree to become a client with my knowledge, we will co-create completely personalized actions based on your goals to move you toward your ideal vision of health within your unique body, lifestyle, preferences, and resources. I practice a holistic approach to health and wellness, which means that I analyze and look at how all areas of your life are connected.

We will discuss the following questions:

- Does stress at your job or in your relationship(s) cause you to overreact?

- Does lack of sleep or low energy prevent you from exercising?

- What Health issues are you experiencing?

- What is your daily water volume intake?

- Are you ready for a change?

DO YOU LISTEN

Reflect on your answer:

_____

_____

_____

_____

As we work together, we will look at how all parts of your life affect your health as a whole. I work with my clients to get in touch with their body's needs because I understand that life happens and your needs will change. I want to equip you with the self-awareness to make the best decisions for yourself in any given circumstance. I believe each person is fully capable of making well-informed decisions as their own expert, not the latest magazine article or fad diet book.

Let's define what you value most from your well-being. We'll use these visions to motivate specific goals that bring you closer to where you want to be. As your coach, I will not dictate a diet for you, but together we will explore why some foods make you feel better than others and how to use that feedback strategically. Together we'll co-create your health goals within reasonable time frames and actionable objectives so that you know exactly what you're working toward. To design your focus with me, register on my website www.thehealthandfitnessadvocate.com and let's get started.

"THERE IS NO PASSION TO BE FOUND PLAYING SMALL - IN SETTLING FOR A LIFE THAT IS LESS THAN ONE YOU ARE CAPABLE OF LIVING."

NELSON MANDELA

CHAPTER 2

LET GO OF SOME WEIGHT

THERE'S A SAYING, "You do better when you know better." So let's get started because I'm getting ready to enlighten you with some knowledge that you may already know, but you may refuse to accept. What's stopping you from changing or making a difference in your life?

What excuses are you prepared to tell:

I drink a lot of water.

Healthy food is too expensive.

Busy schedule.

Gym too expensive.

Don't want to mess up your hair.

I'm fine with my weight.

I'm ok with being Single.

What are your excuses?

Reflect on your answer:

_____

_____

_____

_____

_____

If this is you and you do not want to change, sit back and think how good you will look in the coffin. If you don't wake up and change, you are looking at a few of the following possible future outcomes:

Obesity

Hypertension

Diabetes

Heart Failure

Depression

Loneliness

Cancer

Let's find a way to be healthy and a way to live a better life. Why am I so passionate about Health and Fitness? The reason for this health and fitness journey resulted from my mother dying of Breast Cancer. I really didn't take health or Cancer serious until it hit home in my family. My

LET GO OF SOME WEIGHT

Mother was such a strong role model and a brave soul in her fight with Cancer. She did not want to take Chemo or Radiation because of the pain it would cause, but most of all, the fear of losing her hair and the image she wanted to look at in the mirror. This is why I am so passionate about educating all that will listen to improve their life with simple changes that will make a difference in their future.

When I say, let go of your weight, I am not just talking weight in general, but weight off of your mind and soul allowing you to release stress.

How do you let things go and just forgive to have a healthy life?

Do you experience any anxiety, stress or depression?

Reflect on your answer:

_____

_____

_____

_____

_____

_____

You may not even know that you are depressed. I remember one day while working and sitting in a health clinic waiting to see one of my physicians. There was a pamphlet that had several questions about everyday life situations. The end of the pamphlet included a survey. The results at the end described your current situation/mood. I completed the survey and looked at my score, which was alarmingly high for Depression. I started analyzing my current situation wandering if obesity and depression had a connection because at the time I was at my heaviest, (199 lbs. and a size 16). This was at the time I had broken up with my daughter's father. I was a single mother with no support. I convinced myself that I didn't need him because I was a strong independent woman. I finished work, picked up my daughter from my Mother's house, and completed the nightly routine. Once everything was completed, I searched for my workbag, pulled out the survey and really became extremely emotional. I couldn't stop crying because I knew I was at my heaviest with emotions and actual weight (size 16), which I had a hard time losing after giving birth. I could not understand why losing weight was such a struggle because I was always a size 2. Now I had my answer "Depression," but how do I fix me? I had my pity party for a few days, and then I set out on my journey of getting my life back. Depression was no joke because many people don't understand what the person is mentally going through. You really don't want to be bothered with anyone. You can function with the day-to-day routines, but after that, it's a shutdown. I don't remember feeling sad, but always tired and just wanting to eat, stay at home, and watch TV. The Lifetime channel actually allowed me to cry for what I thought was tears for the characters in the movie, but in retrospect, I was really crying for my situation. I didn't realize I was in depression until I completed the survey because I thought it was just a tired phase I was going through, and I would bounce back soon. Thank God I am the type of person that once I can figure out the problem, then I go into fix it mode. Those of you that cannot bounce back, I beg you to get help from a professional. You have to stop letting people bring you down. You definitely have to learn to give your mind a break by letting go of daily stress. Have happiness during the day by adding laughter and fun to balance your life. Your friends will listen, but will never understand unless they experience the situation.

This takes me back to coping with the loss of my Mother because people try to comfort you, but until you lose a Mother, there's really nothing that you can say that will help a person's emotional state. This is just my opinion, and you may feel different. I know you mean well, but it's a different loss, and there's always a missing link in your heart. I have always connected my weight with my emotional journey.

Do you connect your weight with your emotions?

Reflect on your thoughts:

_____

_____

_____

_____

_____

_____

_____

_____

_____

_____

_____

"Happiness happens on the way to fulfillment."

DR. MARTIN SELIGMAN

Now let's discuss my weight journey that continued from 1993 until I completed my 1st Chicago Marathon in 2002. This was the beginning of my weight loss and my push for a better me because my daughter needed me to be healthy. I pushed and pushed to start improving me, and when I got the control that I desired, I was then able to move on to helping others find themselves. When all is said and done, I realized that sometimes depression and weight are connected, and I believe you can fix them simultaneously. Start asking yourself the following:

What does good health mean to you?

What's your road to good health?

What simple change can you make today?

What will inspire you to want better or do better?

Do you want big results?

Reflect on your answer:

_____

_____

_____

_____

_____

_____

If yes, then you will have to incorporate one small change at a time staying consistent to make it a lifestyle. Now that we have tackled some questions that you will need to answer before you are ready to commit to a healthy you, let's focus on the next connection, which is the body weight that you need to let go. Society labels weight as obesity, fat, overweight or just large. So what is obesity? If you connect obesity with the standard body, mass index society states that obesity is when BMI reaches and exceeds > 30 kg/m or simply overweight is connected to a BMI of > 25 kg/m. According to the latest data from NHANES, one-third of all U.S. adults are considered to be obese and another third is considered overweight.

Why is this acceptable?

Because we don't want to get off the couch and we definitely don't want to eat smaller meal sizes?

Why are we so comfortable with super-sized meals or drinks?

Why are we ok with little to know exercise?

What's wrong with going for a 30-minute walk?

Most people view body fat as relatively harmless and don't mind a little cushion or are just comfortable with the fat because of lack of knowledge. They don't have the desire to look or feel better, but do you know that certain types of dangerous fat is stored around your organs and can also contribute to heart disease, dementia, cancer, depression, and many other diseases? Stored excess body fat and what we have now classified as obesity are actually more than just unsightly. It is downright dangerous and extremely unhealthy. While it is hard to imagine obesity and certain types of body fat as inflammatory diseases of their own, that's exactly what they are.

Ask yourself the following questions:

Why should I change?

How do I change?

Do I want to change?

Can I change for a lifetime?

LET GO OF SOME WEIGHT

Reflect on your answer:

_____

_____

_____

_____

_____

_____

_____

_____

_____

_____

_____

_____

_____

_____

_____

_____

_____

_____

_____

Then try one step at a time because the fat didn't attach to your bodies overnight. I really wanted to emotionally relate to extremely obese people. So I started watching a show titled "My 600-lb. Life," and I have to say each story gave me a new found respect for overweight people. Some really want to get healthy but due to fear and food addiction, they allow lack of love for themselves to hold them back until they reach their rock bottom. I cry whenever I view the television episodes because I know they need support. I want to dedicate my life to giving future support to all that desire a healthy lifestyle.

In my abundance of research, I discovered that about 1 in 3 children are overweight or obese. The studies show that the overweight children are more likely to become overweight adults or obese adults. Obese and overweight people are at risk for diabetes. One key player that has a major role in impacting obesity that affects the rest of the body is leptin. I really had not heard of leptin let alone linking it to obesity then connecting to diabetes because of the risk factors. I don't know if any of you understand the connection, so I wanted to elaborate because knowledge is power. You do better when you know better, right? Leptin is a primary hormone linked to your appetite, which signals feelings of fullness. While leptin actually suppresses the urge to eat, most obese individuals have high blood levels of leptin, which suggests that they are leptin insensitive. Leptin interacts with insulin, and it appears to make the body more sensitive to insulin. Believe it or not, high leptin blood levels are associated with high blood pressure. The more I research, the more I discover that the exact mechanism is not fully understood, but leptin may damage muscle cells. Therefore, it is fair to say that obesity can lead to cardiovascular problems through a number of different pathways.

There are several questions that need to be answered:

- Is your health issue a body weight problem or much deeper?

- Are your eating patterns a significant problem that need to be rectified?

- Are there issues that you are struggling with, which holds you back from the real you?

Reflect on your answer:

_____

_____

_____

_____

_____

_____

_____

_____

_____

_____

_____

_____

_____

_____

_____

_____

_____

_____

_____

_____

_____

_____

If yes, then you will have to start getting things together by accepting your role in each situation. How can you improve yourself with your actions? I am learning to stop and listen more to allow more reaction time. This is definitely a work in progress, and with meditation, prayer, and solitude, you will see improvement. How? I am starting to remove myself from certain situations to allow a better understanding of myself. When you start working on your inner self to get to the root of many issues, you will discover that you will release people, and specific things will be essential. I am not saying it's always you 100% of the time, but I am asking you to realize the part that you play and how to improve you. If this is not fixed normally harboring negativity, fear, or hatred will increase stress. Sometimes we are not even aware of the level in which stress is affecting our health, mind, and body. There was a time in my life that I was so stressed and showing so much outside frustration, but truly internalizing a lot of issues. I was so bad that I became extremely sick and could not eat for 3 months. When I would eat, every part of my body would hurt (excruciating pain). So I discovered that Ginger Ale, Crackers, and Smoothies were the only things that would help. I did that for 3 consecutive months, while visiting several physicians and allowing them to run numerous test. They could not find anything wrong. I just happened to be in church one day and saw my family practice physician. She was extremely nice, and she asked me what was wrong because apparently, I was looking pretty bad. I had lost about 20 - 30 lbs. And I am sure I was looking a hot mess. We discussed my current situation, problems, and overall issues. She prescribed me some pain medications and asked me to eat because I could not take it on an empty stomach. That day is when it all hit me because I had finally taken medication and eaten more than the three items that were consistent on my list, I went to bed because something just didn't feel right. I woke up in the middle of the night in massive pain. I was rushed to the ER to discover that I was having a Gallbladder attack. I needed emergency surgery, but you know me I had to promise that I would come back because I was a single parent and I had to get my daughter in order before I could cater to me. The surgeon allowed me to have the surgery within the next few days. My thought process was, I could go back to the three items on my past list and I would not have any pain. So I organized my daughter and then had my surgery. I was on medical leave from my job for 8 weeks. I came off of medical and quit my job of 14 years on the spot. Why? I knew that 90% of my stress was coming from that job or should I say my Manager at the time. I just knew that I could not go back through that stress, so I prayed and asked God to help me get to my next level of where I should be in my life. I had a job within two weeks of quitting and I truly believe that with faith, favor, prayer, obedience, and listening with an open heart, that God heard me and answered my prayers. I am not telling you to go and quit your job because of stress, but I am saying trust in God and allow him to direct your life. The details are so numerous with this experience of my life that it would take another book to really discuss the details of this situation, emotional baggage, and daily routines that got me through and made me a stronger person today. You must take yourself to a higher level within your soul to grow to your full potential. This will allow your general awareness to increase and your spiritual ear to open to the universe.

"IF YOUR PRESENCE

DOESN'T ADD VALUE,

YOUR ABSENCE WON'T

MAKE A DIFFERENCE!"

ZERO DEAN

CHAPTER 3

TAKE A BREATH

YOU HAVE TO TAKE a deep breath in and release it out allowing you to relax, release stress, help your heart rate, decrease negativity, increase positivity in your life. Get an understanding of how to get control of your blood pressure. Discover different styles of meditation to help with calming your spirit. Hypertension (HTN) also known as high blood pressure is a medical condition in which the blood pressure is consistently increased in the arteries. There are two classifications of high blood pressure; Primary and Secondary. It is known that 90 – 95% of HTN cases are due to the Primary classification. This is due to nonspecific lifestyle and genetic factors. This leaves 5% - 10% remaining, which is considered Secondary due to an identifiable cause that affects the kidneys, arteries, heart or endocrine system. High blood pressure usually does not cause symptoms. So, the next obvious question you want to ask is "What's the cause?"

It's a result of having long-term high blood pressure. This is a major risk factor and a contributor to numerous heart problems and conditions including heart failure, stroke, vision loss, and chronic kidney disease. Statistics show that the lifetime risk of heart failure doubles in people who have a blood pressure greater than 160 mm Hg/90 mm Hg diastolic vs. those that are less than 140/90 mm Hg.

Do you know your blood pressure numbers?

_____

_____

_____

_____

_____

_____

The only way to know (diagnose) if you have high blood pressure (HBP or hypertension) is to have your blood pressure tested. You can go to your physician's office and get your blood pressure checked, but there are blood pressure machines in most grocery stores that are connected with a pharmacy. The most important step for you is to understand your blood pressure numbers and learn how to control high blood pressure.

TAKE A BREATH

What do you know about High Blood Pressure?

_____

_____

_____

_____

_____

_____

_____

_____

_____

_____

_____

_____

_____

_____

_____

_____

_____

_____

_____

Here's a chart of Healthy and unhealthy blood pressure ranges. Learn what's considered normal, as recommended by the American Heart Association.

Blood Pressure Category	Systolic mm Hg (upper #)		Diastolic mm Hg (lower #)
Normal	less than 120	and	less than 80
Prehypertension	120 – 139	or	80 – 89
High Blood Pressure (Hypertension) Stage 1	140 – 159	or	90 – 99
High Blood Pressure (Hypertension) Stage 2	160 or higher	or	100 or higher
Hypertensive Crisis	Higher than 180	or	Higher than 110
(Emergency care needed)			Higher than 110

Note: A diagnosis of high blood pressure must be confirmed with a medical professional. A doctor should also evaluate any unusually low blood pressure readings. Additionally, lower targets may be appropriate for some populations such as African-Americans, the elderly, or patients with underlying issues such as diabetes mellitus or chronic kidney disease.

TAKE A BREATH

Do you know your blood pressure numbers?

Are your numbers in the normal range?

If not, what are you doing about your results besides taking meds to control the high blood pressure?

What's in your refrigerator and Kitchen cabinets?

Are you consistent with exercise?

What are you eating?

Reflect on your answer:

_____

_____

_____

_____

_____

_____

_____

_____

_____

_____

_____

_____

Medications are not the only thing that can help lower your blood pressure. Lifestyle changes such as the list below can lower the risk:

- Weight loss.
- Decrease salt intake.
- Healthy diet.
- Physical exercise.

The 2004 British Hypertension Society guidelines proposed the following lifestyle changes consistent with the US National high BP Education Program in 2002.

Here are a few tips that can possibly help:

- Maintain normal body weight for adults (BMI index 20-25 kg/m2.
- Reduce dietary sodium intake to <100 mmol/day (<6 of sodium chloride or <2.4 g of sodium per day).
- Engage in regular aerobic physical activity such as brisk walking (>30 minutes per day, most days of the week).
- Limit alcohol consumption to no more than 3 units/day for men and no more than 2 units/day for women.
- Consume a diet rich in fruits and vegetables (at least five portions per day).

TAKE A BREATH

Effective use of the above modifications may lower the blood pressure and possible result in you taking one single hypertension medication. Combinations of the above can achieve even better results.

You may not know, but the average person with High Blood pressure can take up to three medications to control their BP. What will you change to make a difference with your blood pressure (Food, Exercise, Stress or Alcohol consumption)?

_____

_____

_____

_____

_____

_____

_____

_____

_____

_____

_____

_____

_____

"Life is ten percent what happens to you and ninety percent how you respond to it."

LOU HOLTZ

CHAPTER 4

GIVE ME SOME SUGAR

WHEN WE THINK OF sugar in the body, the first thing that comes to mind is diabetes. The question that I am now getting a better understanding is how do you know if you have diabetes? In talking to current diabetics, I asked them how they were first diagnosed. They discussed feeling extremely tired, always thirsty, and always going to the restroom to urinate. They still didn't think anything was wrong until they went to the doctor for a regular checkup. When you have an annual routine checkup, there's always blood work ordered. This is when they discovered abnormal levels with their Glucose and A1C levels. If this is describing anything that you are going through, please make an appointment with your Family Practice or Internal Medicine physician and get your blood work completed. When thinking of Diabetes, the first step is to get a basic understanding of the body and how it processes the main culprit of diabetes, which is insulin. Glucose provides the body with its main source of energy, and the pancreas releases the hormone insulin to regulate carbohydrate and fat metabolism and help cells in the liver, muscle, and fat tissue to take up Glucose from the blood, storing it as glycogen in the liver and muscle. In healthy individuals, insulin is released as needed to offset blood glucose; thus more insulin would be released after a meal than after sleeping. When blood glucose falls below a certain level, such as when meals are delayed, the body is not using insulin properly. Insulin resistance means those muscle, fat, and liver cells are not responding properly to insulin and require more than usual to process glucose. Generally speaking, for a person with diabetes or one who is carbohydrate sensitive, a low (slow-releasing) glycemic index food is preferred to a high (fast-releasing) glycemic index food; this helps to keep a steady level of available glucose for your body to use for energy. The glycemic index tells only part of the story. What it doesn't tell you is how high your blood sugar could go when you actually eat the food, which is partly determined by how much carbohydrate is in an individual serving. To understand a food's complete effect on blood sugar, you need to know both how quickly the food makes glucose enter the bloodstream, and how much glucose it will deliver. A separate value called glycemic load does that. It gives a more accurate picture of a food's real-life impact on blood sugar. The glycemic load is determined by multiplying the grams of a carbohydrate in a serving by the glycemic index, then dividing by 100. A glycemic load of 10 or below is considered low; 20 or above is considered high. To help you understand how the foods you are eating might impact your blood glucose level, I have included a glycemic index chart in the back of the book. The chart contains a listing of the glycemic index and glycemic load, per serving, for everyday common foods. At the core of your weight, appetite and mood control are your blood sugar levels, which are controlled largely by insulin. Remember, insulin balances blood sugar levels by bringing them down after we've eaten a high carbohydrate or sugary meal. When we digest food, our body breaks down sugar and starch molecules into simpler units called glucose or fructose. These simple sugars enter our bloodstream and trigger the release of insulin from the pancreas, and then insulin has the important job of ushering blood sugar into cells throughout our body. This process supplies us with energy for things like brain, tissue, and muscular function when it's working properly. At the same time, insulin also corresponds to body fat stores, including the visceral fat stored deep within our bodies. This is why people often call insulin our "fat-storage hormone."

So how do we connect insulin with Diabetes?

What do you know about Diabetes?

_____

_____

_____

_____

_____

We know that insulin resistance does not equal diabetes, but it can lead to type II Diabetes Mellitus (DM). We are aware that 95% of the diabetic population is type II. This occurs when the body either does not make or use insulin correctly. The other 5% is Type I Diabetes population when their bodies produce little or no insulin. Discovering and dealing with the issue of insulin resistance may go a long way in stopping diabetes before it ever evolves. Characteristic symptoms include excessive urine production, excessive thirst and increased fluid intake, and blurred vision. Type I is usually due to the destruction of insulin-producing cells in the pancreas and requiring patients to take insulin; thus, it is called insulin-dependent diabetes. Most develop type I before 30 (juvenile diabetes). Type II- the body becomes resistant to the effects of insulin; this form can often be managed with dietary treatment and medicine. In my research, I found several Diabetic articles that allowed me to get a better understanding and provide facts regarding diabetes. Did you know there are an estimate of 21.1 million Americans >20 years of age having physician diagnosed Diabetes Mellitus (DM)? There are an additional 8.1 million adults with undiagnosed DM, and an almost unfathomable 80.8 million adults with pre-diabetes (fasting blood glucose of 100 to <126 mg/dl). Overall, the prevalence of pre-diabetes in the US adult population is 38%. While I am researching and understanding the information above, I keep asking myself, why don't we do better? What can be done to help educate people to desire a Healthy Lifestyle? Then I realize that this is my purpose in life. I am dedicating my life to help educate and inspire all that will listen and want a Healthy Lifestyle.

Let's start digging deep inside and really take the time to understand the reasons why we make the decisions that we make.

Why can't we get control of the food that we put into our mouth? Why can't we just say NO?

Reflect on your answer:

_____

_____

_____

_____

_____

Stop grabbing for that drink, candy, chips, or dessert?

What is the real problem?

Do you think you are missing a fantastic flavor or sweet that your body just can't do without?

Do you ever connect eating with your current emotions?

Reflect on your answer:

_____

_____

_____

_____

_____

I attend different conferences for my job to increase my educational knowledge to make the right decisions. I find myself getting that piece of bread, glass of wine, and even dessert when I'm out with co-workers. I then equate it to peer pressure or lately just my lack of control because why do I care what they think about me? At the end of the day, this is my body, my life, and my season. Do better when you know better. I always try to justify the "why" behind my decisions.

If I just get real with myself, I need to acknowledge that I am lacking control in that area of my life.

How's your control?

_____

_____

_____

_____

_____

_____

_____

_____

_____

_____

_____

_____

_____

Here are some steps that I take to get control:

- Slowly analyze each situation before I start eating.
- Ask myself specific questions that will connect with my current emotions and listen before reacting.
- Discuss your problems with a nonjudgmental friend.
- Love myself through this journey.
- Train myself to get back on track.
- Be extremely patient.
- Believe in myself "I am a winner."
- Put myself first (Health, Emotions, and Relationships).

Which steps will you try?

_____

_____

_____

_____

_____

_____

_____

_____

_____

_____

_____

"Whatever you hold in your mind on a consistent basis is exactly what you will experience in your life."

ANTHONY ROBBINS

CHAPTER 5

MY HEART IS HEAVY

HOW DOES MY LACK of control with stress, food or wine connect in other areas of my life, like relationships? I find myself praying and asking God for a better understanding and a clear mind with wisdom in order to discern the negativity or wrong people entering my life. Calmness overcomes me when I really connect with the spirit to get to the real issue that I struggle with daily. The connection gives my soul and entire body the peace that I need and desire for improvement. Sometimes I mistaken my struggles with that inner satisfaction thinking that a mate is needed, but in reality, it's desired. The issue of praying for a mate, constantly, but not hearing an automatic answer from God makes me sit back and relax and wait on the blessings that will be coming. I have come a long way with handling no answer from God because I used to be so upset and frustrated. I know that I don't want to spend the remaining of my life by myself. I want to find that special person and spend my life with a partner truly sent by God. I also find myself being very selective. That's the word I would use today, but my friends and family would say that I am too picky. I have my standards and really don't want to settle for any old thing just to have a mate. I desire him to be my soul mate, my best friend and my ride or die. I know that we will have so much in common, but be different at the same time if that make sense to you. My friends know my entire list of requirements and they say that I should not look at his waist circumference or teeth or whatever else and just focus on how he will treat me. I get it, but I know I will spend the remaining of my life trying to change him into that desired mate. I don't want to focus on educating him on why he should lose weight, or eat a certain food or even exercise. I don't want a life partner that has nothing on my list of requirements because I do not want to spend my entire life trying to improve him with certain issues that are considered non-negotiable. That may sound really bad, but I just want to be attracted to my soul mate. I then go into prayer... Lord now you know what he should look like. You know my heart's desire. You know what I have asked for the last ten years. I am still trying to figure out why God will not grant me that prayer. I always justify it by saying that he is just preparing both of us to get ready for a lifetime of happiness. I let each year go by and look at the holidays in disbelief like spending more days alone. This is not a joke anymore, but it happens and I know others are frustrated, but keep praying. Always start the New Year with a positive attitude, clear mind, and set vision. You have to trust that your prayers will be answered. I know that my prayers and desires will come to fruition and I need to stop focusing on what's lacking in my life, but be grateful for all the blessings. I know that I have to prepare myself and make sure that I am ready.

Acknowledge some of your blessings and answered prayers:

_____

_____

_____

_____

_____

_____

_____

_____

_____

_____

"Keep people in your life who truly LOVE you, MOTIVATE you, and make you HAPPY. If you know people who do none of these things, LET THEM GO."

WISDOMLIFEQUOTES.COM

Let's analyze the situation. Have you got your house in order? How does your house look because he may be a neat freak and I am definitely not neat all the time? Then I think will he compromise with a maid? What about my closet, is it ready for a man to move in? I heard someone say to organize your closet and dresser drawers by making room for your mate. Wait a minute, is he suppose to move in or do I move in with him? Does he even have a house or is he renting waiting for a mortgage with his beloved? Can he financially afford a partner or will he come with his half and I have my half? What does his credit score look like? Does he have a school loan? Man this is too much to think about and then I STOP and exhale… maybe single is better. Then I think what if he has an ex-wife, is she nice? How will she accept a new person around her children, because it never fails the ex will never want him until she will see him happy with someone else. Better yet, he better not be a deadbeat dad. Does he see the children and pay for the children? Does he have to go to court because that is a deal breaker? Lord knows I have spent many of my days in child support court trying to get the deadbeat dad to pay for his responsibilities. I definitely did not lay down by myself and end up pregnant because if that was the case, I will just change my name to Mary, right? Get it together, stop exhale. Is being single better?! Get a grip and let's think about the positives. OK… I'm waiting what are they??? He will be my protector, my best friend. He will be a person that I will be able to share my deepest secrets. A person that will be able to lead me into a future we will share. He will take care of me not because I need him to, but because he knows that's his role. He will take the garbage out, clean the car, fill the gas tank, hell even cook because he will love it. Stop and then exhale…. Does he exist and oh yeah let's not forget the best lover ever…. I will need to definitely get myself ready and remove the baggage to make sure that I am ready for this prize, amazing specimen of a man… ladies can you get with that and do you feel what I am saying? How many are in the same boat? How many have tried online dating, blind dates, friend hook-ups, and churchmen?

And NEVER… NEVER ladies are you to go to a married man. I don't care how good it is, what the conversation is and what problems he's having with his wife. Remember, God will never send you someone else's husband. If you think he will, then he may send your husband away when you finally get one. Let's GET a GRIP and stay focused. How do you get yourself together? Let's start from head to toe. How's your mental state with all your past relationships? How's your relationship with your father?

This is where I really struggle because my father was in my life up until I think 10 years old. Then he left and moved on. He would send a card every now and then for holidays or birthdays, but nothing else. When I was much older and had my daughter, I craved that relationship, so I reached out and tried my best to develop a bond. Let me first state that my mother was an amazing lady because she stepped up to be both the mother and father. She did an amazing job; God rest her soul. I'm not saying she was perfect, but she took care of her five children and made sure we didn't lack for anything.

Let's get back to my father because lord knows I have tried, but when I really look at it. I'm as strong as my mother and stubborn as well. I look at it like he wants to be in my life when I don't need him financially or for guidance. Now he needs me, and my pride will not allow me to be there for him. Before you get all on my case, I know what the Bible states, "Honor your mother and your father and your days will be longer." Trust me it's a struggle, and I believe at the beginning of this chapter, I did admit that I was working on it, right? I am writing this book to get control of all connections with Health, Emotions and Relationships to Design my Focus. My issue with my father is that I know that I need to have 'UNCONDITIONAL LOVE" and I have to work on a better relationship …. I am just being real because I'm not bitter or angry or mad. I'm trying to figure out his God given purpose in my life. I need to understand the true connection that I am suppose to have at this point because I have a Godfather that is absolutely amazing and he makes sure that I talk to him every day. I was never comfortable with that idea, and I thought it was the craziest thing because I would get so mad at him. I would say why do I have to talk to you every day? What can we possibly talk about every day? I would get so irritated, but I never realized that's what a father-daughter relationship should be.

My father should be my protector, advisor, and best friend. So that when I meet that Mr. Right, he will mirror my father. This will allow me the peace of mind to understand the real meaning of a Father. This should also enlighten me on the expected treatment of my lifetime partner, soul mate and future husband. Stop. Wait exhale….

What steps will you take to change?

_____

_____

_____

_____

_____

_____

_____

I started analyzing myself while on my book journey and discovered steps to improving my relationship:

- Admit your faults and issues.
- Discuss the problem with the individual.
- Let him/her take some time to soak it in and give you feedback.
- Seek counseling to make sure that you have truly forgiven.

What steps will you try?

_____

_____

_____

_____

_____

I believe we succeed when we pour into our relationship, not when we are constantly taking from them. Always connect in your relationship with helping each other meet goals. The goals should have an individual benefit that will allow success for your partnership. You have to be fully committed to the relationship to expect a stable and long lasting future.

I believe we must envision a Bigger Dream that allows for a true Commitment. Let it go and work on the next area that may need improvement.

"I dream with Powerful Intention. Opening my mind to Spirit, I trust my intuition to deliver powerful visions of my inspired future, and I empower my intent to transform those visions into reality."

JONATHAN LOCKWOOD HUIE

MY HEART IS HEAVY

Now let's get to the main thing that can get you in trouble extremely fast, the "MOUTH." How are the words that come out of your mouth? Are you respectful of yourself as well as others?

Reflect on your answer:

_____

_____

_____

_____

_____

_____

_____

_____

_____

_____

_____

_____

_____

_____

_____

_____

_____

Are you cursing with every sentence and giving the excuse "That's how I've been raised?" My family used that language that's why it's ok. You know that's wrong and you need to reset and try it again. Excuses.... The question is, how do you change it?

_____

_____

_____

_____

_____

I can't tell you to just stop cold turkey because that's not realistic. So take one day at a time and ask your friends/family to try to correct you. Remember, you are cleaning up your mouth for you and your future husband, and the longer it takes, it may take him longer to find you because he's waiting for all the requirements from his list. This is a work in progress and will need your total attention. What if your soul mate has this on the top of his list of requirements? What if he doesn't want a woman with a foul mouth. Maybe he's upset that he hasn't found you, but wait it's too hard for you to clean up your mouth. So you are stuck?

Get it together and pray for deliverance, but also listen more before talking. Take several breaths if someone upsets you before you open your mouth. Try to go into an internal meditation with the full intention of releasing all negativity. Take slow and steady deep breaths bringing positivity in each time. This will calm your soul and spiritual realm to open the doors to peace and blessings.

What have you tried to calm your soul and spirit?

_____

_____

_____

_____

_____

_____

_____

_____

_____

_____

_____

_____

"Say NO to the demands of the world. Say YES to the longings of your own heart."

JONATHAN LOCKWOOD HUIE

Let's now focus on the Physical appearance.

Are you fit, obese, big boned, just needing to tone? Do you exercise on a regular basis and not just once a quarter or right before an event? What do you consider fit because I am not saying that is a size 2 or 4? I get it, but those love handles and that stomach should not be overlapping.

Reflect on your answer:

_____

_____

_____

_____

_____

_____

_____

_____

_____

_____

Let's stop making excuses and just DO IT.

What exercise can you do? Can you join the gym? Can you join the local YMCA? Can you afford a personal trainer? Can you take group classes? Can you join a local walking group? (Join www.dsfit2run.com)

Reflect on your answer:

_____

_____

_____

_____

_____

_____

_____

_____

_____

_____

Whatever it is, get a schedule and do it....

Don't wait for your man to come because he just may walk right passed you because on his list is a fit woman. Keep in mind that you want to get fit for you and love yourself in the process.

MY HEART IS HEAVY

So I want you to get off the couch and stop making excuses. I felt the same at a size 16 with every excuse because I allowed the weight to keep me feeling fatigue and depressed. The crazy part is on my weight loss journey I was more critical of myself because I enjoyed being that size 4. I am always fighting to stay focus on my dream body. Before you get crazy, let me explain what a size 4 is to me. There's no love handles, no back fat and everything fits nice and neat. I can tuck my shirt into my pants and not slightly pull it out to cover the love handles because they show when you wear a fitted shirt.

OHHH yeah, you will need to set an individual goal. So ladies, whatever the goal is, get going, but be realistic.

_____

_____

_____

_____

_____

_____

_____

_____

_____

Men you are not getting off that easy.... Do you really think that looking like you are five months pregnant is attractive? First, it's not healthy, and that's considered visceral fat. Remember, visceral fat was mentioned in a previous chapter connecting it with insulin.

What's visceral fat?

I'm glad you asked. Visceral fat is technically excess intra-abdominal adipose tissue accumulation. In other words, it's known as a "deep" fat that's stored further underneath the skin than "subcutaneous" belly fat. It's a form of gel-like fat that's actually wrapped around major organs, including the liver, pancreas, and kidneys. Men if you have a protruding belly and large waist, that's a clear sign that you are storing dangerous visceral fat. While it's most noticeable and pronounced in obese individuals, anyone can have visceral fat, many without even knowing it. Visceral fat is especially dangerous because, as you'll find out, these fat cells do more than just sit there and cause your pants to feel tight — it also changes the way your body operates.

Carrying around excess visceral fat is linked to an increased risk for:

- Coronary heart disease
- Cancer
- Stroke
- Dementia
- Diabetes
- Depression
- Arthritis
- Obesity
- Sexual dysfunction
- Sleep disorders

Visceral fat is considered toxic and spells double-trouble in the body because it's capable of provoking inflammatory pathways, plus signaling molecules that can interfere with the body's normal hormonal functions. In fact, it acts almost like its very own organ since it's capable of having such a large impact on the body. Fat cells do more than simply store extra calories. They have proven to be much more involved in human physiology than we had previously thought. We now know that fat tissue itself acts like its own organ by pumping out hormones and inflammatory substances. Storing excess fat around the organs increases production of pro-inflammatory chemicals, also called cytokines, which leads to inflammation. It also interferes with hormones that regulate appetite, weight, mood, and brain function. Having a lean belly is a key indicator of health, so your body tries to preserve this by controlling your appetite and energy expenditure. To prevent dangerous fat buildup, the body basically works like an orchestra of chemicals that tells us when to eat and when we are full. This chemical feedback system, which is built on communication between the brain and other major organs — a.k.a. the brain/body connection — is what's responsible for either keeping us at a healthy weight or making us more susceptible to weight gain and visceral fat storage. Everyone knows someone especially those who are sedentary, chronically stressed, or maintain an unhealthy lifestyle.

How will you change with this information?

_____

_____

_____

_____

_____

_____

_____

A different type of fat (subcutaneous fat), which builds up under the skin, has less of a negative impact on health and is easier to lose than visceral fat. In fact, excessive deposits of visceral fat are associated with many serious health problems including: cardiovascular disease, Type II Diabetes, and High Blood Pressure. These are the very topics that we have discussed in previous chapters. How do you gain this fat because you look great and out of nowhere this fat appears? Right? People gain abdominal fat for a variety of reasons, including eating foods high in fat and sugar as well as maintaining an inactive lifestyle. People tend to get heavier and heavier as time goes on — and one of the main reasons is that stored body fat affects hunger levels, especially visceral fat. It might seem hard to imagine, but your existing stored fat is largely governed by your metabolism. Fat messes with our appetites and makes it easier to overeat due to hormonal changes that take place. Higher levels of insulin also promote more efficient conversion of our calories into body fat, so this vicious cycle continues. Eating refined carbohydrates, as opposed to complex carbohydrates in their natural state like vegetables and fruit, can cause the body's "set point" for body weight to increase. Your "set point" is basically the weight that your body tries to maintain through control of the brain's hormonal messengers. When you eat refined, carbohydrates such as white flour and sugar, the fat-storing hormones are produced in excess, raising the set point and making it hard to follow a moderate-calorie, healthy diet. This is why it's important to kick your sugar addiction and address weight gain and visceral fat formation early on, as opposed to letting the situation escalate.

What can make the fat accumulate quicker?

_____

_____

_____

_____

_____

_____

I'm glad you asked because not exercising for long periods of time is one of the answers. A little exercise daily can greatly inhibit the development of visceral fat. Keep in mind there are other issues such as: lack of proper sleep, constant stress or an uncontrollable such as aging. People tend to lose muscle mass as they age resulting in higher body fat. Instead of trying to figure out how much of your visible belly fat is visceral and how much is subcutaneous, just realize that any big belly, love handles, and large waistline poses a risk and is unhealthy. Women with a waist circumference that's more than 35 inches and men with a waist circumference more than 40 inches are at increased risk for various diseases and should try to lower fat stores as soon as they can. Research allows for a better understanding of the connection with the different types of body fat. The visible jiggly fat that we envision daily is known as white fat or white adipocytes. The main purpose is to store energy and release hormones into the blood stream. White fat can be stored in two different places, which is in both visceral or subcutaneous fat.

You're more likely to lose visceral fat when you do a combination of exercising and eating right, which are both important for hormone regulation.

According to Dr. Josh Axe

Stop. Wait and exhale….

Steps to improving that Physical appearance:

- Physicians recommend a minimum of 30 minutes of aerobic activity like brisk walking (Hence local walking group) or jogging at least four times a week.

- Stomach exercises, like sit-ups, build muscle in the area, but will not reduce this fat.

- Resistance training with bands or gym equipment, this will help subcutaneous fat, but not abdominal fat. Aerobic exercise can have a significant impact on visceral fat, which may show results for up to a year after any weight loss occurs.
- Improve your diet with heavy fruits and vegetables **(Ask me about JuicePlus)**, high fiber foods and lean meat (If you are not a vegetarian of course).

Do you think you could ever consume a whole food based nutrition lifestyle of 30 fruits, vegetables and grains daily?

MY HEART IS HEAVY

Let me know your thoughts:

_____

_____

_____

_____

_____

_____

_____

_____

What steps will you try?

_____

_____

_____

_____

_____

_____

_____

_____

_____

_____

The bottom line is you have to make this a Lifestyle change and not a quick fix.

Remember, smoking and excessive drinking can lead to increased visceral fat. So you will need to do these in moderation or STOP all together. Also keep in mind that meditation, Yoga, Pilates, and prayer has proven to be successful because all relieve stress. Now that you have some tips to improve your physical appearance, let's move to another area.

We discussed the mouth and what comes out of your mouth. Now let's discuss the inside of your mouth. Let's work on the next area by opening your mouth and looking inside. What's in your mouth and how do your teeth look when you smile? Are you satisfied with your smile? If the answer is no, then fix the teeth and please explain to me why you can eat all of that unnecessary food, drinks, and whatever, and not take great care of your teeth.

_____

_____

_____

_____

_____

_____

Let's start with answering the following questions:

- Do you correctly brush your teeth daily?
- How often do you floss?
- Do you have an appointment with your dentist twice a year, which is every 6 months?

Reflect on your answer:

_____

_____

_____

_____

_____

_____

If not why are you waiting because I know you want to kiss once you meet your soul mate, right? Not if those teeth are jacked, stacked, and discolored because there are so many procedures out here now that can help you get, straight, clean, healthy and white teeth. Start with making an appointment with your dentist. If you need recommendations, I will be happy to send you some connections. I will talk to my dentist and have him on standby as well as to give referrals. He's amazing, and I have gone to the same dentist for 21 years. I have referred several of my friends and just strangers that I have met at various places. When you go on a regular basis, your teeth and gums are healthy… let's get going because here's a list of things that can happen if you don't take care of your teeth. According to Columbia University College of Dental Medicine. Some cardiovascular (heart and artery) disease may affect your oral health. It also may require changes in your dental treatment and how you receive dental care. One disease that I am familiar with because I was diagnosed with it in the past is periodontal disease.

Symptoms of periodontal disease include:

- Persistent bad breathe.
- Red, swollen or tender gums.
- Gums that bleed when you brush your teeth.
- Gums that pull away from the teeth.
- Loose teeth.
- A change in the way your teeth move when you bite down.

Heart attacks can sometimes feel like pain that starts in the chest and spread to the lower jaw. Other times it may be pain that starts in the jaw or in the left arm or shoulder. Your physician will tell you how long you should wait for a dental appointment after a heart attack.

MY HEART IS HEAVY

Keep in mind that some medications that you take may change the way that your dentist can treat you (i.e. blood thinning medicines, high blood pressure medications, or cholesterol medications to just name a few.)

What   medications   are   you   taking?

_____   _____

_____   _____

_____   _____

_____   _____

_____   _____

Are you seeing any improvements?

_____

_____

_____

_____

_____

_____

_____

Let's discuss the next area that might need improvement. The feet because I have heard from several guys that this is a deal breaker. Well, you want the woman to wear high heels to look sexy for you, but do you realize the damage that they put on our feet. Believe me, I love my Jimmy Choos and I always make sure that they are extremely comfortable before I walk out of the store. The top of the line shoes must be comfortable at all time or leave them in the store because the pain is just not worth it. We all love them, but guess what, the damage done to your feet is just not good. When you really focus on your feet and analyze the extent of the damage. You may discover, the damage could have resulted from your childhood issues with wearing tight shoes, and that's another issue.... Please research a Podiatrist and make the appointment to get in there to get help. I am currently researching the best physicians for me, but will not have any surgeries until I complete my 3rd Chicago Marathon in October 2017. I am definitely not satisfied with my feet because I want them to look a certain way in my sandals. I am so self conscious that every time I wear sandals I feel that everyone's looking at my feet. I know it's my insecurities and I have to work through my issues one step at a time. I acknowledge my dislike and I move on to a plan to fix it for me. I can honestly say though, I met my soul mate years ago, and the love of my life took one look at my feet and didn't care. He said that's just runners' feet. So this wasn't a deal breaker for him. There were other issues. So again, if you are not satisfied with what your feet look like, get them fixed. Once I get my feet fixed, I will post a before and after but not before... Lord.

Share your thoughts regarding your imperfections that keep you stressed:

_____

_____

_____

_____

_____

This will allow you to release any negative thoughts and move to positive universe.

"FAILURE ISN'T FATAL, BUT...FAILURE TO CHANGE...MIGHT BE!"

JOHN WOODEN

CHAPTER 6

GET IT TOGETHER WITH BALANCE

LET'S FOCUS ON HEALING the rough insides allowing a growth process with softening the internal body to balance from inside out. There will be a glow that others will see that illuminates from you and allows the attraction of powerful people and situations to surround you. Always remember that God will put people in your life for a reason or a season. I now add for a lesson or a testimony.

Here's an interesting situation that I recently encountered: So I am on vacation in Jamaica, and I met this guy that looked pretty depressed. We were in a buffet setting and ended up meeting up at every station. I think it was a coincidence, but who knows that maybe it was the Lord wanting me to hear his story. I finally spoke and said, "Do we like the same food or are you following me?" He smiled and of course blamed it on the food. We began to talk, and it was apparent that we were supposed to meet because he had just lost both of his parents within the last eight months and was really sad. He used this as a getaway and left his family and friends to be by himself because he just could not take the loneliness. I then realized that was my story 12 years ago when I traveled to Italy and Paris to just get away. I told him that my getaway started with the loss of my Mother, but it blossomed into a beautiful time that I now spend with my daughter Brittanie. The time that we travel allows for great bonding time and improving our Mother-Daughter relationship along with our great friendship. I also spend a lot of time in prayer and meditation along with reflecting on my mother and actually realize how much I miss her and wish that she was still alive. So I believe the Lord wanted me to meet him and give him encouragement that it will get better in due time, but it's okay to mourn in your own way and time. Food for thought, everyone wants to console you at the time of mourning and it does help, but for me, it escalates the memories, which makes me sad. I now know that I have to focus on the good memories to allow for laughter and just to remember how blessed I was to have my Mother for 59 years as opposed to others that had their loved ones for a shorter time.

Reflect on some of your good memories:

_____

_____

_____

_____

_____

_____

_____

_____

_____

_____

_____

The emotional loss is one of the hardest to get passed. We all know that everyone has to go eventually. The problem is when we think that person has been taken too soon. I guess my struggle is "what's too soon?" What's our definition of too soon? We all want that question answered from God so that we can get a better understanding or answer to "WHY?"

When I ask people if this is true, they all agree and they just don't have the answer and unfortunately will never have it until it's our turn. We will then know, but will not be able to tell the people here on earth.

My mother would always say if she ever had a chance to come back and help her children, she would in a heartbeat. She wanted to make sure that her death was not in vain. She wanted us to know that she loved us that much that she would come and help us in any way possible. It has been over 12 years, and I have seen her a few times in my dreams, but not having a clear understanding of the purpose. I know the very first time that she appeared to me when I was in Rome it was confirmation. She let me know that I was exactly where I was supposed to be at that time. I have found myself really meditating, seeking wisdom with a desire for a clear mind. I have experienced so many emotions while on my book journey. I now believe that counseling will definitely help and in the midst of writing this book, I have researched different counseling options. I stay in constant prayer, meditation, and just getting better connected to God to know my purpose and understand the reasoning behind my passions to get people healthier. I know this is exactly where God wants me. I know that my desire to want people to be at their comfort level is lead by God. I know this has to be a lifestyle and not a diet. I want people to be able to go everywhere in the world and continue with their day-to-day healthy lifestyle.

I know this will take time because you have to clean up your lifestyle before you can really focus on being healthy. I am not saying that you should get rid of everything. I want you to have a realistic mindset, a balanced perspective, and a better understanding of the choices that you make with everything.

Reflect on your lifestyle and the Simple changes you will incorporate:

_____

_____

_____

_____

_____

_____

_____

_____

_____

_____

You need to have a conversation with yourself on why do I want this food, drink or to just sit on the couch?

Reflect on your answer:

_____

_____

_____

_____

_____

_____

_____

Will it have a positive or negative impact on my body?

Reflect on your answer:

_____

_____

_____

_____

_____

_____

_____

What's the real reason for wanting it?

_____

_____

_____

_____

_____

_____

Is it for pure pleasure or am I feeling stressed, depressed, sad, and need something to relieve the pressure?

Reflect on your answer:

_____

_____

_____

_____

_____

_____

_____

_____

So, will you allow the emotions to get you down, or how will you fix it from this point?

Write down your thoughts:

_____

_____

_____

_____

_____

_____

_____

_____

_____

_____

_____

_____

_____

_____

_____

_____

_____

_____

Please utilize the FOUR pillars that help me everyday:

Prayer

Counseling

Meditation

Exercise

CHAPTER 7

GETTING PAST EMOTIONAL SCARS

WE ALL HAVE SOME type of emotional baggage that holds us back from true connections. We have to dig deep inside and discover that exact moment in time we allowed it to impact our mind, spirit, and soul. Once you pinpoint the issue, it will take courage, dedication and a clear mind to work through the problem. The process will take courage to confront your fears, courage to forgive the person or people that hurt you, and finally, courage to love yourself through the pain to healing and moving into your true universe of happiness and joy. When I discussed this topic with several of my girlfriends, I discovered that we all share similar stories, especially with family connections. I also discovered that a lot of us handle things in a similar manner, but there are a few that really handle their issues with a spiritual connection to allow God to intercede and take control. In the past, I have really tried to pray through my situations, but in my humanness, I have failed several times allowing my anger to take control. While writing this book, I am really processing all of my emotions and allowing God to work through me and keep me in my peaceful place. Keep in mind that some of your friends and family may not be able to handle the light that God has given you or the path that you are destined. Keep in mind that your light is so bright, some people cannot handle your success, and they do not understand your passion. You have to realize there will be some negativity that will require you to walk away and get your clarity back.

It is ok to take a break and ask the following:

- Do I have the will to change?
- Will my change result in happiness and peace?
- Can I awaken my power to resolve the issues?
- Do I have the energy to sustain the time to resolve the issues?
- What is the ultimate barrier that's stopping my growth to happiness?
- Can I maintain the change and make it a Lifestyle?

Reflect on your answer:

_____

_____

_____

_____

_____

_____

_____

_____

_____

_____

_____

_____

_____

_____

_____

_____

_____

_____

_____

_____

_____

"The less you respond to negative people, the more peaceful your life will become."

ZIGLARFAMILY.COM

I have taken a sabbatical from all negativity while completing this book because I believe God is giving me clarity, patience, a forgiving heart, and the spirit of discernment to grow within allowing happiness and joy to settle in my mind, body, and soul. I understand that sometimes in life people do not want to see you always happy and successful because of their lack. When you give up your happiness, you give people power over you, and that should never happen in your life. Understand the power that you have within and design your focus for a better you. I now understand that the true key to a life full of happiness and joy is "FORGIVENESS." When we allow ourselves to truly forgive the person of their actions is when we return to our anointed spiritual center.

The first step is to let go of your ego and do not let anyone affect you.

Do not let anyone into your inner being. Nothing should takeaway your happiness.

GETTING PAST EMOTIONAL SCARS

Who do you need to forgive?

_____

_____

_____

_____

_____

_____

_____

_____

_____

_____

_____

_____

_____

_____

CHAPTER 8

FORGIVENESS IS KEY

I TRULY BELIEVE THAT forgiveness harbors bitterness because of past hurts. The past can really instill anger, resentment, and frustrations to allow it to take over your life and internalize situations. According to Wikipedia, FORGIVENESS is the intentional voluntary process by which a victim undergoes a change in feelings and attitude regarding an offense, let go of negative emotions such as vengefulness, with an increased ability to wish the offender well. When you break it down, you must let go. Remember, when you forgive, it's for you not for the other person because it allows you to heal and opens up your blessings. You have to stop processing all of the bad memories of others actions or lack of actions toward you. You have to truly forgive them by forgetting all the wrong and truly loving them in the place that you are at the particular moment. You will never change the outside until you improve the inside.

FORGIVENESS IS KEY

Let it go, and believe me, I know it's really hard to dig deep and discover the choices you have to make in life that will allow you true happiness.

The biggest problem is your follow through. You have to fully let go of the bitterness that you hold in your heart and grow into a positive state of mind that nothing anyone will attempt to negatively impact you will hold any space within your universe. So many people will say I will forgive you, but I will never forget. Is that true forgiveness? Do you feel that once you say it that makes it 100%, but what are your actions? When that person approaches you, can you look at them and really embrace them like nothing ever happened in the past. If you cannot, then the forgiveness is not completed.

Why is it so hard to forgive?

What are the real issues that we go through that will not let us let it go?

Reflect on your answer:

_____

_____

_____

_____

_____

_____

_____

_____

_____

_____

_____

_____

_____

_____

_____

_____

_____

_____

_____

_____

_____

FORGIVENESS IS KEY

I struggle with this every day and this is exactly why I put a forgiveness chapter within this book. I really want to get past this problem in my life so that I can truly be free from all the bitterness, hurt, and ugliness. I do not accept this anymore from people and I am really pushing to eliminate it out of my life. I ask myself every day, what can I do to change and how do I get through this because it can be with strangers, friends, co-workers and family? I think we really hold on to these feelings with the people that we are closer to because we see them more often. We also did not select them into our lives and we are forced to maintain that relationship. God put us together for a reason, and we have to get along. We definitely select our friends and can decide to let them go at any time especially when it's so negative and disruptive. I am sure there is a place that you can meet in the middle and begin the process to forgiveness for you and the other person. I use to always think it's the other person and they are aware of how they are treating me. I now pretend like I am in the other person's shoes and I ask myself the following:

- Do you understand how mean, hurtful, and pure hateful you appear? Are you intentionally trying to hurt me?

- Are you in such a bad place in your life that you want everyone to be "miserable?"

I really want the person to trade places and let them see exactly how they are treating the other person. I have been hurt in my past by friends, family members, and strangers, but I ask myself NOW, how do I want to handle it? Think about how you handle it?

Reflect on your answer:

_____

_____

_____

_____

_____

_____

_____

In the past, I would lash out and act as ignorant as they appear, but now I take a sabbatical from the person. I want to make sure that it's not me provoking them to act out of line. I want to make sure that I give myself enough time away to allow both parties to reflect on their actions. I want them to wonder why I'm all of a sudden too busy for them. It's not that I don't want to be bothered, it's that I want to get my mind right along with my soul to make sure that when I step back into their life, I am relaxed and patient with the ability to tolerate them. I do not want to remember the past or expect them to act crazy, but I am aware of their past actions because of experiences.

I now try to analyze myself regarding my actions:

- How will I positively handle the next interaction?
- How can I practice meditation or breathing to allow a positive universe around me at all times?
- How can I stay in a happy place within my life and help them to feel better about themselves?
- How do I get rid of the anger that I harbored from their past actions and their disruptive lifestyle?
- How do I decrease my stress level by improving my reaction and helping me get to a better place?

Reflect on your answer:

_____

_____

_____

_____

_____

_____

Do you get what I'm saying because sometimes it's not about you, they are just extremely unhappy, and they want you to be at their level? If you really believe that you want to improve, seek the answers to the questions every day of your life. You will realize that the person that is giving you the most grief and negativity just doesn't know better and sometimes they don't mean any harm. Allow them to get it out, but always remember, DO NOT ACCEPT WHAT THEY SAY INTO YOUR SPIRIT.

"Desire is the key to motivation, but it's determination and commitment to an unrelenting pursuit of your goal - a commitment to excellence - that will enable you to attain the success you seek."

MARIO ANDRETTI

So here's what I consider a funny story:

I went to church one Sunday morning, and my Pastor preached a fantastic sermon. He said that people would come at you and put all type of negative things into your spirit and/or life, but it's up to you to NOT accept that into your spirit. I listened to the message and really understood the deep meaning of the message. I left church feeling energized, blessed, and just overwhelmed by the life that God has blessed me to have and live. I went to a family member's house, and I found myself suddenly in a sit-down intervention. They proceeded to tell me that I was cold, heartless, and nobody in the family wanted to talk to me. That people are scared to talk to me because of my negative vibe. I stopped the intervention and said what my pastor had stated in the church. I truly want to listen to you, but I want to let you know that I am listening, but I will not accept that into my spirit because that's not me. I was feeling good with taking the message from church and applying it directly to my life. The only problem was, the people telling me this message didn't accept it very well and thought I was rebelling and not wanting to listen. We agreed to disagree and then I realized that we are all different and we should NOT judge each either, but love everyone just like Jesus. So now I exhale and really take time to celebrate my life and all of my blessings that God has bestowed on me and I feel so grateful. I am happy, excited, and extremely motivated to live the best life with helping others achieve their Lifestyle Balance.

According to pathos.com, there are 6 steps that can help you find forgiveness:

1. Forgive with a desire to let go and have no revenge.

2. Make a plan - this will allow you to free up energy to work on you to regain as much of what was lost or taken from you.

3. Stop dwelling and retelling - We always want to keep telling everyone about our hurtful experiences thinking that might change our situation. If you want to tell someone, I would suggest you seek counseling to allow true professional help to get you on the right track to proper forgiveness.

4. Seek grace because without God's grace it may be extremely difficult to heal some wounds or hurtful events. If, after meditation and prayer then consultation, you find that there really is nothing you can do to reclaim what was lost or taken from you, focus your energy on developing new goals that will help you reconstruct a compelling future.

5. Read the book, "The Life God Wants You to Have": Discovering the Divine Plan When Human Plans Fail it can be a tremendous help for figuring out what God is calling you to work toward in the next chapter of your life.

6. Seek Professional Help - allowing your faith to help heal with talking through issues with God and a professional. This will allow you to discuss your feeling of bitterness, resentment, anger or any other emotions that are holding you back from true happiness.

FORGIVENESS IS KEY

How will you work on your forgiveness?

_____

_____

_____

_____

_____

_____

_____

_____

_____

_____

_____

_____

_____

_____

_____

_____

_____

_____

_____

"*Our deepest fear is not that we are inadequate. Our deepest fear is that we are powerful beyond measure. It is our Light, not our darkness, that most frightens us.*"

MARIANNE WILLIAMSON

CHAPTER 9

LET'S GET GOING

THERE IS A NEED FOR you to design your focus in every aspect of your life. Here are some universal steps you should consider:

- Seek Counseling
- Talk to someone you trust
- Feel your emotions (Fear, Anger, Emptiness, etc.)
- Love your Body
- Love yourself

There are so many planners that can help you get organized in ALL areas of your life. I believe that checklists should be a beginning step to planners. I am including a few of my checklist in this book to help you get focused, gain clarity, and organize your life for a healthy balance. Let's start building our list to initiate planning your goals for each day, week, month, and finally the entire year. I want you to be well prepared for this NEW YOU and set all goals possible. I truly believe in planning, whether it's for your Health, Emotional, or Relationships, it will help you improve all aspects of your life.

Which area will you work on first?

_____

_____

_____

_____

_____

_____

_____

This will allow you to identify your goals, motivations, and appointments rather they are daily, weekly, monthly or yearly to enable you to connect all things necessary for an organized and balanced life.

What are your goals?

_____

_____

_____

_____

_____

_____

_____

_____

_____

What are your trigger points that promote bad habits keeping you stuck in the same position and not allowing growth?

_____

_____

_____

_____

_____

_____

What behaviors will you need to improve during the planning stages?

_____

_____

_____

_____

_____

_____

Make sure that you fill out the goals and accomplishments for each area.

Health:

_____

_____

_____

_____

_____

Relationship:

_____

_____

_____

_____

_____

Emotional baggage:

_____

_____

_____

_____

_____

"A great paradox of life is that while we must create plans for our future in order to live a joyful life, simultaneously, we must graciously accept whatever events life actually throws against us. If we fail to plan, we merely bob helplessly - like a cork on the sea of life. If we resist whatever life delivers to us, we create untold misery for ourselves. Only by charting our course, and then continuously recharting that course in response to the events of life, can we achieve success and happiness."

JONATHAN LOCKWOOD HUIE

Here are a few tips to help with your planning expectations:

Health is the most important for you to make and keep updated. You will need to list all of your health issues if there are any, all medications currently taking along with dosage, all physician appointments, and the nature for each visit, vitamins and/or supplements currently taking and the reasons. Comment section to confirm a clear understanding of your test results and the next steps if they are abnormal. Comment section to have a clear plan for follow-up and improvement.

Relationship should be in a planning position because we spend time on everything else, but do not keep our mind open, prepared and ready for our mate. We say we are ready, but are we 100% ready? Do you have your HOUSE in order to receive your mate? Let's plan to always be ready for the mate that God has aligned to our future. You have to know what type of person you want in your life and what type of person you are attracting based on your overall aura. You will need to have a daily, weekly, and monthly log that will help you decide which is best for you. You will also need a plan to eliminate bad behaviors or remove consistent issues that hold you back from love.

Emotional baggage that we all have can be an extreme struggle within ourselves because we rationalize the outcomes. We justify the reasons why we should do the things like stop talking to a certain person or just not involving them in your life. We figure if we don't see them then it's good. The problem is when we see them, and if it stirs up emotional issues within you, then that's a problem. You have to clear the environment around you so that it will remain positive and pleasant at all times regardless of who enters your worldly space. Have you ever had an issue with a person and your friends knew about it, so they tried not to allow the connection to take place? I believe the Lord will test you and let you bump into that person to make you realize that you have issues inside that need to be fixed. When you see that person, it's so awkward, you feel angry, frustrated or even mad, but if you stop and take a deep breath, and visualize your planner with next step possibilities, you will realize that you are on the right track. You have to believe in yourself and allow every future situation to result in positivity. Why? Because you are moving in the right direction with consistent positive behavior and a pleasant attitude at all times. You are so proud of yourself, right? Well, let me tell you from firsthand it's a work in progress and please take one day at a time to make sure you release all bitterness and emotional baggage.

So, use the following checklists and let's get the best you possible. This will allow you time to work on your healing and improve the new you!!!

What are your thoughts?

_____

_____

_____

_____

_____

_____

_____

_____

_____

_____

_____

_____

"TO GO AGAINST THE DOMINANT THINKING OF YOUR FRIENDS, OF MOST OF THE PEOPLE YOU SEE EVERYDAY, IS PERHAPS THE MOST DIFFICLUT ACT OF HEROISM YOU CAN PERFORM."

THEODORE H. WHITE

Health Checklist

TYPE		Date Completed	Recommendation
	OBGYN Visit		Every 3 years
	Mammogram		Annual
	Prostate Exam		Annual
	Colonoscopy		Every 10 years
	Dental Exam		Every 6 months
	Eye Exam		Annual
	Flu Shot		Annual
	Routine Physical (Weight, Labs)		Annual

My Goals

My Motivations

My Medications

	WEIGHT	BLOOD PRESSURE	GLUCOSE	FLU SHOT	STRESS LEVEL	CHOLESTEROL
Before						
After						

Relationship Checklist

www.thehealthandfitnessadvocate.com

TYPE		Date Completed with Notes
	ANALYZE SELF	
	ANALYZE PAST RELATIONSHIPS	
	REPAIR BAD BEHAVIORS	
	INTRODUCE MEDITATION	
	ORGANIZE HOUSEHOLD	
	PREPARE SELF FOR A RELATIONSHIP	
	CONNEECT FRIENDSHIP	
	CONFIRM YOUR SPIRITUALITY	

My Goals	My Habits	My Concerns

My Relationship Struggles

	FEAR	LISTENING ISSUES	COMMUNICATION	ANGER	FORGIVENESS	TRUST
WITH ME						
WITH PARTNER						

Design YOUR Focus

Emotional Checklist

www.thehealthandfitnessadvocate.com

TYPE		Date Completed with Notes
	ANALYZE SELF	
	FACE TO FACE DISCUSSION	
	PROFESSIONAL CONSULTATION	
	MEDITATION	
	ACTIVITY TO INCREASE POSITIVITY	
	UNDERSTAND YOUR TRIGGERS	
	CONNECT YOUR TRIGGERS WITH EMOTIONS	
	BALANCE YOUR EMOTIONS TO CONENCT WITH HAPPINESS	

My Goals   **My Habits**   **My Concerns**

My Emotional Baggage

	FEAR	BITTERNESS	PAIN	ANGER	FORGIVENESS	STRESS
WITH ME						
WITH OTHERS						

117

GLYCEMIC CHART

	GLYCEMIC INDEX (GLUCOSE =100)	Serving size (Grams)	GLYCEMIC LOAD PER SERVING
BAKERY PRODUCTS AND BREADS			
Banana cake, made with sugar	47	60	14
Banana cake, made without sugar	55	60	12
Sponge cake, plain	46	63	17
Vanilla cake made from packet mix with vanilla frosting (Betty Crocker)	42	111	24
Apple muffin, made with rolled oats and sugar	44	60	13
Apple muffin, made with rolled oats and without sugar	48	60	9
Waffles, Aunt Jemima®	76	35	10
Bagel, white, frozen	72	70	25
Baguette, white, plain	95	30	14
Coarse barley bread, 80% kernels	34	30	7
Hamburger bun	61	30	9
Kaiser roll	73	30	12
Pumpernickel bread	56	30	7
50% cracked wheat kernel bread	58	30	12
White wheat flour bread, average	75	30	11
Wonder® bread, average	73	30	10
Whole wheat bread, average	69	30	9
100% Whole Grain® bread (Natural Ovens)	51	30	7
Pita bread, white	68	30	10
Corn tortilla	52	50	12
Wheat tortilla	30	50	8
BEVERAGES			
Coca Cola® (US formula)	63	250 mL	16
Fanta®, orange soft drink	68	250 mL	23
Lucozade®, original (sparkling glucose drink)	95	250 mL	40
Apple juice, unsweetened	41	250 mL	12
Cranberry juice cocktail (Ocean Spray®)	68	250 mL	24
Gatorade, orange flavor (US formula)	89	250 mL	13
Orange juice, unsweetened, average	50	250 mL	12
Tomato juice, canned, no sugar added	38	250 mL	4

GLYCEMIC CHART

	GLYCEMIC INDEX (GLUCOSE =100)	Serving size (Grams)	GLYCEMIC LOAD PER SERVING
All-Bran®, average	44	30	9
Coco Pops®, average	77	30	20
Cornflakes®, average	81	30	20
Cream of Wheat®	66	250	17
Cream of Wheat®, Instant	74	250	22
Grape-Nuts®	75	30	16
Muesli, average	56	30	10
Oatmeal, average	55	250	13
Instant oatmeal, average	79	250	21
Raisin Bran®	61	30	12
Special K® (US formula)	69	30	14
GRAINS			
Pearled barley, average	25	150	11
Sweet corn on the cob	48	60	14
Couscous	65	150	9
Quinoa	53	150	13
White rice, boiled, type non-specified	72	150	29
Quick cooking white basmati	63	150	26
Brown rice, steamed	50	150	16
Parboiled Converted white rice (Uncle Ben's®)	38	150	14
Whole wheat kernels, average	45	50	15
Bulgur, average	47	150	12
COOKIES AND CRACKERS			
Graham crackers	74	25	13
Vanilla wafers	77	25	14
Shortbread	64	25	10
Rice cakes, average	82	25	17
DAIRY PRODUCTS AND ALT.			
Ice cream, regular, average	62	50	8
Ice cream, premium (Sara Lee®)	38	50	3
Milk, full-fat, average	31	250 mL	4
Milk, skim, average	31	250 mL	4
Reduced-fat yogurt with fruit, average	33	200	11

GLYCEMIC CHART

	GLYCEMIC INDEX (GLUCOSE =100)	Serving size (Grams)	GLYCEMIC LOAD PER SERVING
FRUITS			
Apple, average	36	120	5
Banana, raw, average	48	120	11
Dates, dried, average	42	60	18
Grapefruit	25	120	3
Grapes, black	59	120	11
Oranges, raw, average	45	120	5
Peach, average	42	120	5
Peach, canned in light syrup	52	120	9
Pear, raw, average	38	120	4
Pear, canned in pear juice	44	120	5
Prunes, pitted	29	60	10
Raisins	64	60	28
Watermelon	72	120	4
Baked beans	40	150	6
Black-eyed peas	50	150	15
Black beans	30	150	7
Chickpeas	10	150	3
Navy beans, average	39	150	12
Kidney beans, average	34	150	9
Lentils	28	150	5
Soy beans, average	15	150	1
Cashews, salted	22	50	3
Peanuts	13	50	1
PASTA and NOODLES			
Fettucini	32	180	15
Macaroni, average	50	180	24
Macaroni and Cheese (Kraft®)	64	180	33
Spaghetti, white, boiled, average	46	180	22
Spaghetti, white, boiled 20 min	58	180	26
Spaghetti, whole-grain, boiled	42	180	17
SNACK FOODS			
Corn chips, plain, salted	42	50	11
Fruit Roll-Ups®	99	30	24
M & M's®, peanut	33	30	6
Microwave popcorn, plain, average	65	20	7
Potato chips, average	56	50	12
Snickers Bar®, average	51	60	18

GLYCEMIC CHART

	GLYCEMIC INDEX (GLUCOSE =100)	Serving size (Grams)	GLYCEMIC LOAD PER SERVING
VEGETABLES			
Green peas	54	80	4
Carrots, average	39	80	2
Parsnips	52	80	4
Baked russet potato	111	150	33
Boiled white potato, average	82	150	21
Instant mashed potato, average	87	150	17
Sweet potato, average	70	150	22
Yam, average	54	150	20
MISC.			
Hummus (chickpea salad dip)	6	30	0
Chicken nuggets, frozen, reheated in microwave oven 5 min	46	100	7
Pizza, Super Supreme (Pizza Hut®)	36	100	9
Honey, average	61	25	12

The complete list of the glycemic index and glycemic load for more than 1,000 foods can be found in the article "International tables of glycemic index and glycemic load values: 2008" by Fiona S. Atkinson, Kaye Foster-Powell, and Jennie C. Brand-Miller in the December 2008 issue of <u>Diabetes Care</u>, Vol. 31, number 12, pages <u>2281-2283</u>.

Image: © Amarosy | <u>Dreamstime.com</u>

Updated: August 27, 2015 Originally published: February 2015

One Final Thought

LOVING THE OLD YOU TO GET TO THE NEW YOU

Here are a few questions that you will need to ask yourself to awaken the LOVE for the old you and connect the LOVE to the new you.

What does good health mean to me?

What's my selected pathway to good Health?

What simple change will I implement for my big results?

What will it take to love myself?

Do I have the hunger or desire to change?

What triggers my negativity?

Do I experience any anger that I need to release?

What motivate me to change?

What main area will require my immediate attention to design my focus?

Write down your thoughts:

_____

_____

_____

_____

_____

_____

_____

_____

_____

_____

_____

_____

_____

_____

_____

_____

What do you think about Alkaline water?

Do you believe that Alkaline water will help?

What are your thoughts about an Acid pH body vs. Neutral pH body or Alkaline pH body?

Write down your thoughts:

_____

_____

_____

_____

_____

_____

_____

_____

_____

_____

_____

_____

ABOUT THE AUTHOR

Deana Patterson MBA, CMR, BCCL, known as the Health and Fitness Advocate, founder and president of her nonprofit organization DSFIT2RUN, Inc., is the author of Design your Focus. She is an Integrative Nutrition Health Coach with a clear passion that allows her to dedicate her life to providing education for those interested in designing their focus for a healthier Lifestyle. She is committed to providing personal health coaching and improving the emotional connection to help you return to that spiritual center. She has been called to share her health experience with over 25 years in the pharmaceutical industry and life tools that bridges her enthusiasm for growth and development. She believes that everyone has potential that will result in true happiness with everyday living. She also believes that everyone has a calling that will connect their passions with their dreams.

She is a graduate of the Institute for Integrative Nutrition where she learned innovative coaching methods, practical lifestyle management techniques, and over 100 dietary theories – Ayurveda, gluten-free, Paleo, raw, vegan, macrobiotics, and everything in between. Her education has equipped her with extensive, cutting-edge knowledge in holistic nutrition, health coaching, and prevention. Drawing on her expertise, she works with clients to help make lifestyle changes and choose health-promoting ways that produce real and lasting results. She helps you develop a deeper understanding of food and lifestyle choices that work best for you, improving your energy, balance, health, and happiness.

She will have discussions beyond food, seeking to bring balance to important elements of your life such as love and relationships, as well as career and money. She will personally and carefully guide you to make simple, small changes that transform your life. With individual and group coaching sessions, she will find the ideal setting and space that will help you achieve your personal goals. Each session will leave you feeling inspired and motivated.

Deana would like to connect and help you design your focus for a better you.

www.thehealthandfitnessadvocate.com

Facebook: DSFIT2RUN

Deana Patterson

Instagram: DSFIT2RUN

Nonprofit: www.dsfit2run.com

Juice Plus: www.wpatterson.juiceplus.com

NOTES:

_____

_____

_____

_____

_____

_____

_____

_____

_____

_____

_____

_____

_____

_____

_____

_____

_____

_____

_____

_____

_____

_____

_____

Design YOUR Focus